The Big Book of Pressure Cooker Dessert Recipes

Easy, Inspired Dessert for Eating Well

Willie S. Duvall

Sommario

Introduction

The Ninja Foodi multi-cooker is among the devices that everybody should have in their cooking area. The tool can replace 4 little pieces of equipment: slow cooker, air fryer, pressure cooker and dehydrator.

This recipe book consists of a few of the recipes we have tried with the multi-cooker. The dishes vary from breakfast, side meals, fowl, pork, soups, seafood, desserts, as well as pasta. Furthermore, we've put together lots of vegan dishes you ought to attempt. We created these dishes taking into consideration novices which's why the food preparation procedure is organized. Besides, the recipes are tasty, enjoy reading.

DESSERTS

Dump Cake

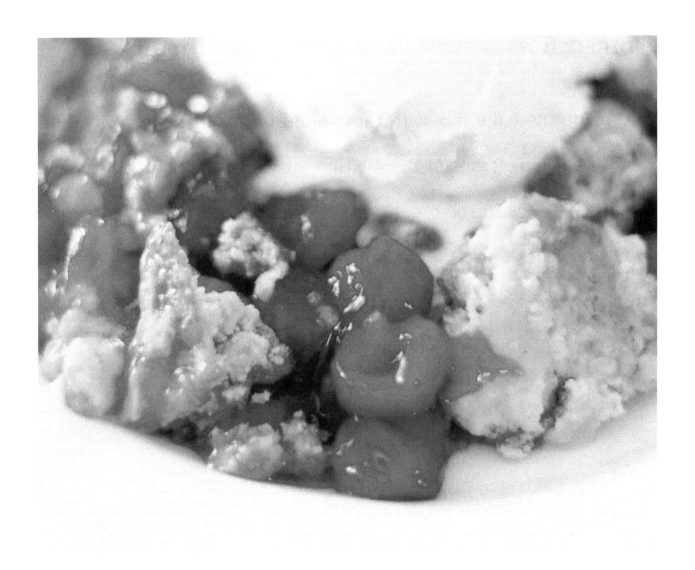

INGREDIENTS (6 Servings)

3 tablespoons of butter, melted

2 cups of cake mix

1 can of pie filling

DIRECTIONS (PREP + COOK TIME: 30 MINUTES)

Combine the cake mix with the melted butter in a bowl. Stir and add the filling. Transfer the mixture into a baking pan and cover it with a foil. Insert the reversible rack and place the pan containing batter into it. Close the Crisping lid and preheat the Foodi on bake mode over 325°F for two minutes. Once preheated, cook the dump cake for 25 minutes. Cool it and serve in slices.

Pressure Cooked Apples

INGREDIENTS (4 Servings)

4 apples, cored

1 1/2 cup of water

1/2 cup of sugar

1/2 cup of dates, roughly chopped

1/4 cup of walnuts or raisins, roughly chopped

2 tablespoons of Goji berries

1 teaspoon of cinnamon powder

DIRECTIONS (PREP + COOK TIME: 15 MINUTES)

Cut off the bottom and top of cored apples. Place them in the Foodi and add water, sugar, nuts, dates, Goji berries, and cinnamon. Close the pressure lid and cook on high mode for 10 minutes. Let the accumulated steam release naturally and open the lid.   Serve your cooked apples with the cooking liquid.

Easy Applesauce

INGREDIENTS (4 Servings)

3 pounds of apples

1/4 cup of sugar

1/2 cups of apple juice

Pinch of salt

1/2 teaspoon of ground cinnamon

1/2 teaspoon of ground cardamom

1 tablespoon of freshly-squeezed lemon juice

DIRECTIONS (PREP + COOK TIME: 14 MINUTES) Peel the apples, remove the cores, and slice them. Combine all the ingredients and close the pressure lid. Cook the apple mixture on high mode for 4 minutes. Quick release the in-built steam and open the lid. Puree the mixture using an immersion blender.

Chocolaty Rice Pudding

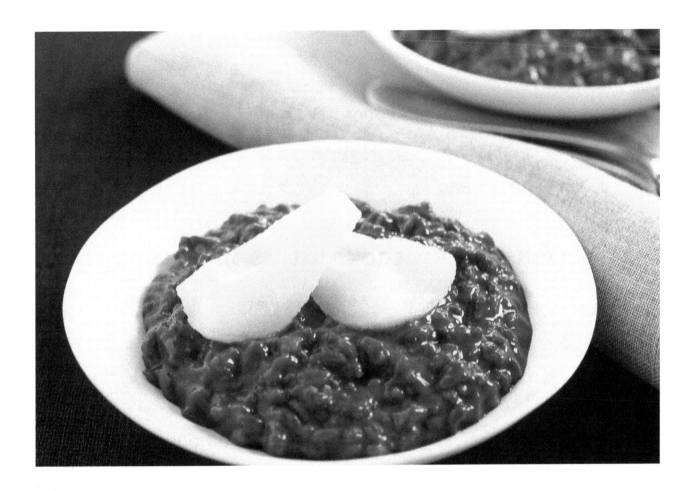

INGREDIENTS (5 Servings)

A cup of rice, uncooked

1/2 cup of sugar

2 tablespoons of butter

2 tablespoons of cocoa powder, unsweetened

1 teaspoon of vanilla flavor

2 cups of milk ,½ cup of evaporated milk

A cup of water , 1 egg

DIRECTIONS (PREP + COOK TIME: 19 MINUTES) Melt butter
on sauté mode. Add the rice, milk, and water. Stir and add vanilla,
cocoa, and sugar. Stir thoroughly and leave it clump- free. Close
the pressure lid and cook the butter mixture on high mode for 14
minutes. Quick release the in-built steam and open the lid. Mix
the evaporated milk and egg in a small bowl. Add a half cup of the
hot rice pudding and mix. Add another ½ cup of the rice pudding
and stir. Stir and transfer the mixture into the Foodi pot. Sauté it
for2 minutes or until it thicken.

Candied Lemon Peels

INGREDIENTS (30 Servings)

6 organic lemons, top and bottoms cut off and peeled

3 cups of sugar, divided

6 cups of water, divided

DIRECTIONS (PREP + COOK TIME: 40 MINUTES) Add the lemon peels to the Foodi. Add 4 cups of water and close the pressure lid. Cook the lemons on high mode for 3 minutes. Let the pressure exit naturally for ten minutes and quick release the rest. Drain water and rinse the lemon peels with cold water. Rinse the pot and add the rinsed lemon peels, 21/2 cups of sugar and the remaining water. Set your Foodi to sauté mode and cook-stir your lemon for 5 minutes to melt the sugar. Close the pressure lid and cook on high mode for ten minutes. Let the pressure exit naturally and open the lid. Transfer the peels on a parchment paper and let it cool for twenty minutes. Spread the remaining sugar over a wide plate and toss the cool lemon peels with it. Shake off excess sugar. Put the sugary peels on a sheet pan and chill for 6 hours. You can put it into glass jars and refrigerate for 2 months. Enjoy with coffee or use as a garnish for cakes.

Hot Peach and Blackberry Cobbler

INGREDIENTS (6 Servings)

4 cups of sliced peaches, frozen

2 cups of frozen blackberries

Zest from a lemon Juice from 2 lemons (1/3 cup juice) 2/3 cup of sugar

A teaspoon of ground cinnamon

5 tablespoons of cornstarch

2 cups of water

For the Topping:

1 1/2 cups of flour

1 tablespoon of ground cinnamon

A cup of light brown sugar, packed

1/4 teaspoon of kosher sea salt

1 1/2 teaspoons of vanilla extract

2/3 cup of unsalted butter, melted

DIRECTIONS (PREP + COOK TIME: 30 MINUTES)

Mix the blackberries with the sliced peaches in a baking pan. Combine the lemon zest with the fresh lemon juice, cornstarch, sugar, and a teaspoon of cinnamon in a bowl. Pour the mixture over the pan content and stir. Set aside for 10 minutes. Place the pan on the rack and pour some water in the pot. Fix the rack in the Foodi and close the pressure lid. Cook the lemon mixture on high mode for 7 minutes. Meanwhile, combine the flour with the brown sugar, a tablespoon of cinnamon, and salt in a bowl. Stir well. Add the butter and vanilla and stir. Allow the in-built pressure to exit naturally for 10 minutes and quick release the rest. Open the lid and add the fruit mixture. Let it rest for 15 minutes as it thickens. Spread the toppings over the fruit mix and close the crisping rid. Air-crisp the cobbler at 350°F for 10

minutes. Cool and serve with frozen vanilla.

Egg Leche Flan

INGREDIENTS (4 Servings)

½ cup of white sugar

2 tablespoons of water

4 large eggs

A can (12 oz) of evaporated milk

1 can (14 oz) of sweetened condensed milk

1 teaspoon of lemon zest

1 1/2 glasses of water

DIRECTIONS (PREP + COOK TIME: 25 MINUTES)

Combine sugar with water in a bowl. Stir. Microwave the mixture for four minutes and avoid burning it. Remove and transfer the mixture to a ramekin or pan. Combine the eggs with evaporated milk, condensed milk, and lemon zest in a bowl. Transfer the mixture into a ramekin or pan Add water to the Foodi pot and insert the rack in it. Place the ramekins on the rack and close the pressure lid. Cook the mixture on high mode for ten minutes. Let the accumulated steam exit naturally for ten minutes and quick release the rest. Open the lid and remove the rack. Drain excess fluids on the flan using a paper towel and chill for 12 hours.

Strawberry Jam

INGREDIENTS (5 Servings)

1 cup of raw honey

1 pound of organic strawberries, diced

DIRECTIONS (PREP + COOK TIME: 20 MINUTES)

Melt the honey on sauté mode and add the strawberries. Boil until they turn pink. Close the pressure lid and cook on high mode for 3 minutes. Let the pressure exit naturally and open the lid. Mash the cooked strawberries and boil the cooking fluid on sauté mode. Pour your strawberry jam into a jar ready for use.

Citrus Canola Cake

INGREDIENTS (8 Servings)

4 eggs

1 cup of canola oil

A cup of sugar

1 orange, juice and zest

1 lemon, juice and zest

A tablespoon of baking powder

1 cup of all-purpose flour

1/4 teaspoon of kosher salt

Powdered sugar, for garnishing

DIRECTIONS (PREP + COOK TIME: 50 MINUTES)

Combine the eggs with canola oil, sugar, juices, and zests in a food processor. Pulse well. Mix the flour with baking powder and salt in a mixing bowl. Add the salted baking into the mixer and pulse. Grease an 8- inch baking pan with oil and add butter. Place the buttered pan on the rack. Close the crisping lid and bake over 325°F for 3minutes.   Pour the puree in the pan and close the crisping lid again. Bake the puree over the same temperature for 40 minutes. Remove the pan from the Foodi and allow the cake to cool for around 15 minutes. Garnish your citrus canola cake with powdered sugar.

Vanilla Cake

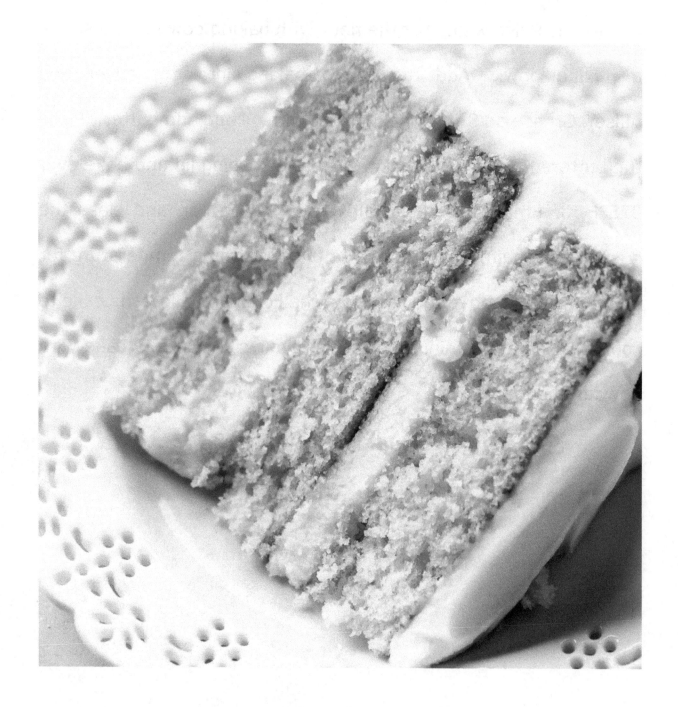

INGREDIENTS (6 Servings)

1 ½ cups of pie filling

1 ½ glasses of cake mix

½ tube of melted vanilla frosting

2 eggs

DIRECTIONS (PREP + COOK TIME: 60 MINUTES)

Grease a baking pan with the cooking spray. Combine the cake mix with eggs in a bowl and fold the filling in it. Transfer the mixture to pan and cover with foil. Fix the reversible rack and place the pan containing the cake mix on it. Close the Crisping lid and preheat the Foodi on bake mode over 325°F for two minutes. After that, bake your vanilla cake over the same temperature for 50 minutes.

Peach Cobbler

INGREDIENTS (6 Servings)

1 box (15.25-oz) of white cake mix, divided

6 peaches (peeled and sliced)

¼ cup of softened butter

DIRECTIONS (PREP + COOK TIME: 25 MINUTES)

Put half of the dessert mix in a large bowl. Add the butter and mix well. Arrange the peaches on a multi-purpose pan and sprinkle them with the cake butter mix. Cover the mixture with foil and place it on a reversible rack. Insert the pan in the rack and close the crisping lid. Bake your peach cobbler over 550°F for thirty minutes.

Blueberry Pancake Muffins

INGREDIENTS (6 Servings)

A cup of all-purpose flour

1 1/2 teaspoons of baking powder

1/4 teaspoon of baking soda

2 teaspoons of sugar

1/4 teaspoon of salt

3/4 cup of buttermilk

1 tablespoon of canola oil

1 egg

3 tablespoons of canned blueberries, drained

1 1/2 cups of hot water

Cooking spray

DIRECTIONS (PREP + COOK TIME: 40 MINUTES)

Combine the flour with the baking powder, baking soda, salt, and sugar in bowl. Mix the buttermilk with oil and eggs in another bowl. Combine the buttermilk mixture with the flour mixture. Add the blueberries and stir. Treat a 6-cup muffin pan with cooking spray and spoon the batter into the muffin cups. Pour water into the pot and insert the rack. Place the pan containing butter on the rack and close the crisping lid. Bake the batter over 350 °F for 25 minutes.

Mango Cheesecake

INGREDIENTS (2 Servings)

1 can (14-oz) of sweetened condensed milk

¼ cup of mango puree

1 cup of Greek yogurt

DIRECTIONS (PREP + COOK TIME: 38 MINUTES)

Grease a pan with nonstick cooking spray. Mix the remaining ingredients in a bowl and transfer them to a coated pan. Cover the pan with aluminum foil and put it in a rack. Add water to the Foodi pot and fix the rack containing a yogurt mix. Close the pressure lid and cook on high mode for 30 minutes. Release the in-built pressure naturally for 20 minutes and quick release the rest. Cool the cheesecake on a wire rack for 5 hours. Top it with the mango puree and garnish with cardamom powder or nuts.

Baked Apples

INGREDIENTS (4 Servings)

2 apples (halved, core removed, but skin intact)

4 teaspoons of light brown sugar

Juice from a lemon

1/4 cup (1/2 stick) of butter, cut in 16 pieces

8 teaspoons of granulated sugar

DIRECTIONS (PREP + COOK TIME: 50 MINUTES)

Pierce the apple halves 6 times. Put the crisper plate in the basket and fix it in the Foodi. Preheat the unit on air fry mode on 325°F for 3 minutes. Cover both the basket and the plate with a foil and squeeze apple pieces around the foil (cut side up.) Sprinkle with brown sugar and lemon juice, top with butter. Air-fry the apples over the same temperature for 45 minutes. Half way, remove the basket and sprinkle the apples with sugar. Cook until softened and serve with your preferred toppings.

Peach Dump Cake

INGREDIENTS (6 Servings)

2 cans (15-oz) of peaches with juice

1 teaspoon of ground cinnamon 1/4 cup of butter, cut into pieces

1/2 box of vanilla cake mix A cup of water

DIRECTIONS (PREP + COOK TIME: 30 MINUTES)

Pour the halved peaches into a greased baking pan. Add the cinnamon and stir. Squeeze the cake mix in the peaches and swirl. Set the butter slices over the cake mix. Pour some water into the Foodi and insert the rack into it. Place the greased pan on the rack and cover it with foil. Close the pressure lid and cook on high mode for 25 minutes. Quick release the accumulated vapor and open the lid. Close the crisping lid and broil your dump cake for 5 minutes. Cool and serve.

Cranberry Oat Bars

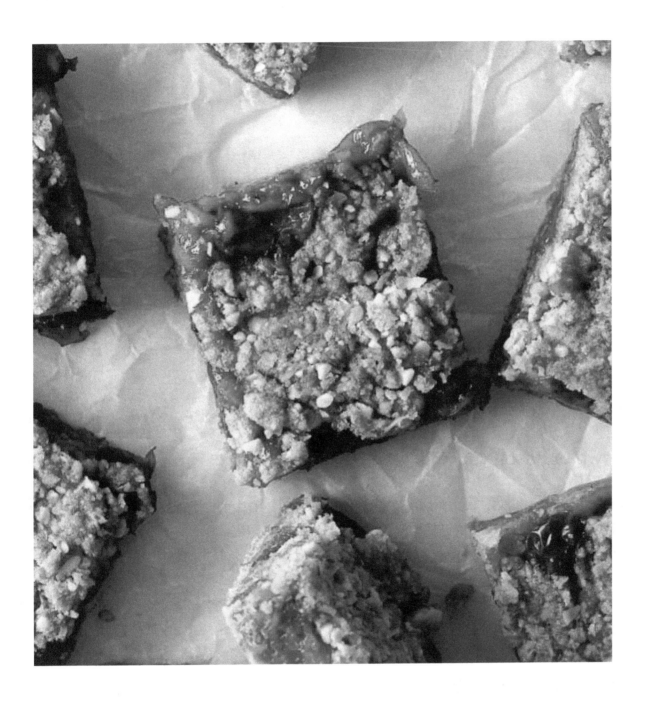

INGREDIENTS (8 Servings)

1 cup of all-purpose flour

1 cup of rolled oats, quick-cooking

1/4 teaspoon of baking soda

1/3 cup of brown sugar

1/2 cup (1 stick) of butter, room temperature

1 cup of whole cranberry sauce

DIRECTIONS (PREP + COOK TIME: 40 MINUTES)

Combine the flour with oats, baking soda, and brown sugar in a bowl. Add butter and blend using a pastry cutter until it forms coarse crumbs. Close the crisping lid and preheat the Foodi unit on bake mode over 325 °F for 5 minutes. Press the mixture over a greased 8 inch pan (Set aside 1 cup). Spread the cranberry sauce over the crumb mix. Close crisping lid and bake on same temperature for 30 minutes. Remove, cool, and cut into bars.

Pumpkin Pie Pudding

INGREDIENTS (6 Servings)

2 eggs

1/2 cup of heavy cream

3/4 cup of sweetener

1 teaspoon of pumpkin pie spice

15 oz of canned pumpkin puree

1 teaspoon of vanilla extract

DIRECTIONS (PREP + COOK TIME: 40 MINUTES)

Whisk the eggs with the remaining ingredients and pour the pumpkin mixture into a greased pan. Add water to the Foodi pot and insert the rack. Place the greased pan on the rack and cover it with a foil. Secure the pressure lid and cook on high mode for 20 minutes. Let the in-built steam exit naturally for 10 minutes and quick release the rest. Open the lid and drain all the water from

the pudding. Refrigerate your pie pudding for at least 7 hours and

serve with the whipped cream.

Apple Dumplings

INGREDIENTS (8 Servings)

8 oz (1 can) of crescent rolls

1 large Granny Smith apple

4 tablespoons of butter

1/2 cup of brown sugar

A teaspoon of ground cinnamon

1/2 teaspoon of vanilla extract

A pinch of ground nutmeg

3/4 cup of apple cider juice

DIRECTIONS (PREP + COOK TIME: 20 MINUTES)

Core the apples, peel, and cut it into 8 wedges. Preheat the Foodi

unit and open the rolls. Roll the dough flat and the apple wedges in crescent rolls. Melt butter in a pot and add the sugar, cinnamon, vanilla, and nutmeg. Stir. Put the dumplings in the Foodi and drizzle with the apple cider. Close the pressure lid and cook on high mode for 10 minutes. Let the accumulated steam exit naturally. Allow your apple dumplings to cool and serve, while drizzled with cider syrup and sugar.

Easy Pumpkin Puree

INGREDIENTS (10 Servings)

3 1/2 to 4 lbs of pie pumpkin

1 cup of water

DIRECTIONS (PREP + COOK TIME: 30 MINUTES)

emove the pumpkin stem. Fix the rack on your Foodi and put a cup of pumpkin in it. Close the pressure lid and cook the pumpkin on high mode for 12 minutes. Let the accumulated steam exit naturally and open the lid. Transfer the cooked pies of a cutting board and slice into two. Take your seeds and peel the skin off. Blend the slices to a puree and refrigerate.

Upside-Down Cheesecake

INGREDIENTS (4 Servings)

2 packages (8 oz each) of creamy cheese

2 large eggs

2/3 cup of sugar

1 teaspoon of vanilla extract

1 cup of water

2 tablespoons of melted butter

1/2 package (8 oz) of sandwich cookies, of preference

Chocolate, caramel, or strawberry syrup

DIRECTIONS (PREP + COOK TIME: 65 MINUTES)

Combine the sugar with cream cheese in a mixing bowl. Add the vanilla and eggs. Stir. Pour the sugar mixture into a 7- inch greased pan and cover with a foil. Pour water and fix the steam

rack in the Foodi. Cook the mixture on low mode for 35 minutes.

Let the pressure exit naturally for 15 minutes and remove the

foil. Set it aside for thirty minutes and refrigerate for at least two

hours. Pulse the cookies and melted butter and cover the cooled

cheesecake with it. Drizzle the cake with the strawberry syrup and

refrigerate for 30 minutes.

Mexican Pot du Crème

INGREDIENTS (6 Servings)

1 1/2 cups of heavy cream

1/2 teaspoon of ground cinnamon

2 tablespoons of coffee-flavored liqueur

1/4 teaspoon of chili powder

1/4 cup of sugar

5 egg yolks

A pinch of kosher salt

2 bars of bittersweet chocolate, melted (4 oz each)

1 cup of water

DIRECTIONS (PREP + COOK TIME: 20 MINUTES)

Preheat the Foodi unit on sauté mode and add the milk, heavy cream, cinnamon, liqueur, and chili powder. Whisk the egg yolks, sugar, and salt in a large bowl and add the warm cream mix, whisking gently. Whisk the melted chocolate and share it between six ramekins. Wrap each ramekin with a foil. Add water to the pot and fix the rack in it. Place the ramekins on the rack and stack the rest on top. Close the pressure lid and cook on high mode for 8 minutes. Let the in-built steam exit naturally for 10 minutes and quick release the rest. Remove the ramekins using tongs, remove the foil, chill, and serve the crème with whipped cream, if desired.

Baked Spice Cookies

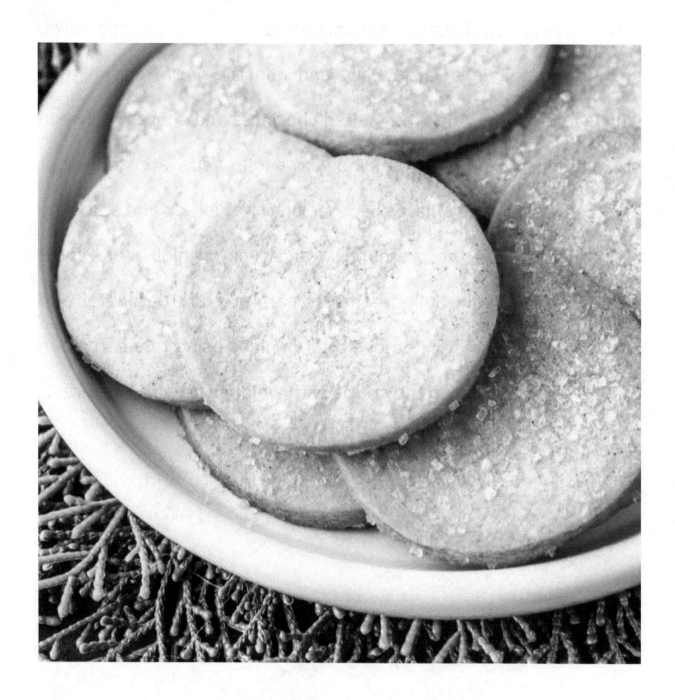

INGREDIENTS (18 Servings)

2 ½ cups of almond flour

½ cup of sugar

4 tablespoons of butter, softened

2 tablespoons of water

A large egg

1 teaspoon of ground cinnamon

2 teaspoons of ground ginger

1 teaspoon of baking soda

¼ teaspoon of salt

½ teaspoon of ground nutmeg

DIRECTIONS (PREP + COOK TIME: 25 MINUTES)

Mix the butter with sugar, egg, and water in a blender. Puree well. Combine the flour with cinnamon, ginger, baking soda, salt, and nutmeg in a bowl. Add the puree to the bowl content. Roll some balls from the mixture and place them on a lined baking pan.   Close the crisping lid and bake the balls over 350°F for fifteen minutes or until the cookies' tops turns slightly brown.

Pumpkin Bread Pudding with Apple–Vanilla Sauce

Ingredients for 8 servings:

Non-stick cooking spray 1 ½ cups 2% milk 2 eggs ¾ cup canned pumpkin ¼ cup sugar plus 1 tbsp sugar, divided 3 tbsp light butter with canola oil divided 1 tsbp Pumpkin Pie Spice 2 tsp vanilla extract divided ⅛ tsp salt 8 oz multigrain Italian loaf bread torn into small pieces 1 ¼ cups Water 1 sheet aluminum foil 18 inches long ¾ cup apple juice 1 ½ tsp cornstarch

Directions and total time – 1-2 hours

• **Coat a 7 inch nonstick springform pan with cooking spray.** • **Whisk together the milk, eggs, pumpkin, ¼ cup of the sugar, 2 tbsp of the light butter, the pumpkin pie spice, 1 tsp of the vanilla extract, and salt in a large bowl until well blended. Add the bread cubes and toss to coat well. Let stand for 10 minutes to allow the bread to absorb the milk mixture, stirring occasionally. Place the bread mixture into** the springform pan; press down on the bread with the back of a spoon. • Place the water and a trivet in the Instant Pot. Cover the springform pan entirely with foil. Make a foil sling by folding an 18 inch-long piece of foil in half lengthwise. Place the pan in the center of the sling and lower the pan into the pot. Fold down the excess foil from the sling to allow the lid to close properly. • Seal the lid, close the valve, and set the Manual/Pressure Cook button to 40 minutes. • Use a natural pressure release for 10 minutes, followed by a quick pressure release. When the valve drops, carefully remove the lid. Remove the pan and sling carefully using the ends of the foil. Remove the foil from the springform pan. Let stand for 15 minutes to cool. • Meanwhile, remove the trivet and discard the water in the pot. Whisk together the apple juice and cornstarch in a small bowl. Press the Cancel button and set to Sauté. Then press the Adjust button to "More" or "High." Add the juice mixture and the remaining 1 tbsp of sugar to the pot. Bring to a boil and boil for 1 minute, or until thickened, stirring constantly. Remove the insert from the Instant Pot, and stir in the remaining 1 tbsp of light butter and 1 tsp of vanilla extract. • Cut the bread pudding into 8 wedges and serve topped with the sauce.

Chocolate and Banana Chip Cake

Ingredients for 8 servings:

½ cup coconut oil room temperature 1 cup monk fruit sweetener 2 large eggs room temperature 3 medium bananas mashed 2 cups oat flour 1 ½ tsp baking soda ½ tsp salt ½ cup stevia-sweetened chocolate chips

Directions and total time – 1-2 hours

• In a large bowl of a stand mixer with a paddle attachment, add the oil, sweetener, and eggs and beat together on medium speed until well combined. • Add the mashed banana and beat until combined. • Add the flour, baking soda, and salt and beat again until combined. • Remove the paddle attachment and stir in the chocolate chips. • Spray a 6 inch Bundt cake pan with cooking oil. Transfer the batter into the pan. Place a paper towel over the top of the pan and then cover with aluminum foil. • Add 1 ½ cups water to the Instant Pot inner pot and then place a steam rack inside. Place the Bundt pan on the steam rack. Secure the lid. • Press the Manual or Pressure Cook button and adjust the time to <strong<="" strong="">. </ strong • When the timer beeps, let pressure release naturally for 10 minutes, then quick-release any remaining pressure until float valve drops, then unlock lid. • Allow to cool completely before removing from pan and slicing to serve.

Steel Cut Baked Oatmeal Bars with Raspberry

Ingredients for 6 servings:

3 cups steel cut oats 3 large eggs 2 cups unsweetened vanilla almond milk ⅓ cup erythritol ¼ tsp salt 1 cup frozen raspberries 1 tsp pure vanilla extract

Directions and total time – 1-2 hours • **In a medium bowl, mix together all ingredients except the raspberries. Once the ingredients are well combined, fold in the raspberries. • Spray a 6" cake pan with cooking oil. Transfer the oat mixture to the pan and cover the pan with aluminum foil. • Pour 1 cup water into the Instant Pot and place the steam rack inside. Place the pan with the oat mixture on top of the rack. Secure the lid. • Press the Manual or Pressure Cook button and adjust the time to 15 minutes. • When the timer beeps, quick-release pressure until float valve drops and then unlock lid. • Carefully remove the pan from the** inner pot and remove the foil. Allow to cool completely before cutting into bars and serving.

Mango and Sticky Rice

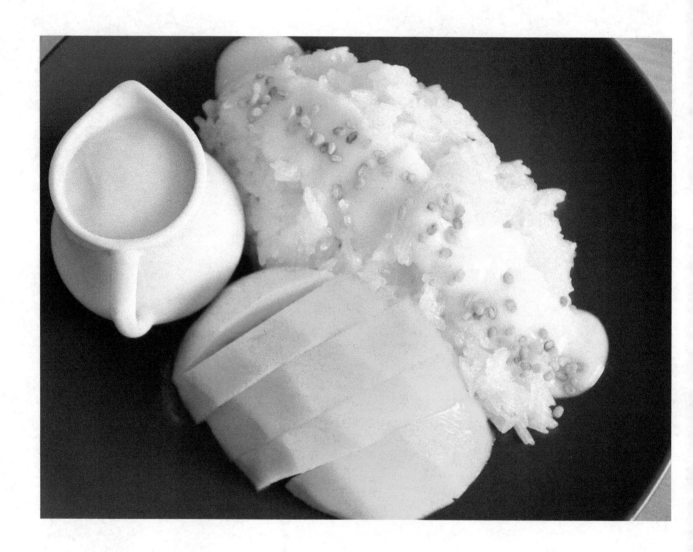

Ingredients for 4 servings:

1 cup Thai sticky rice sweet rice, or glutinous rice 1 ⅓ cups

canned full-fat coconut milk well stirred 7 tbsp organic cane sugar ½ tsp fine sea salt or kosher salt plus more to taste 1 tbsp cornstarch 2 ripe Ataúlfo mangoes peeled, pitted, and thinly sliced or diced, honey, about 6 ounces each 2 tbsp yellow mung beans toasted, or 2 teaspoons toasted white sesame seeds or black sesame seeds

Directions and total time – 30-60 min

• **For easy removal of the pan from the Instant Pot, create a foil sling. (Alternatively, you can use oven mitts to carefully remove the pan.) • Place the sticky rice in a large bowl and add water to cover. Gently stir the rice with your hands, then drain the water, and repeat 4 or 5 times until the water runs almost clear. This removes the excess starch and prevents the rice from becoming gummy. Place the rinsed rice in a heatproof glass or stainless steel bowl that fits inside the inner pot of your Instant Pot. Add ⅔ cup cold water to the bowl to cover the rice. • On the counter, place the bowl on top of the steamer rack with the handles facing up and arrange the foil sling (if using) underneath the** steamer rack. Pour 1 ½ cups water into the inner pot of the Instant Pot. Carefully lower the steamer rack and bowl into the inner pot using the foil sling or steamer rack handles. • Secure the lid and set the Pressure Release to Sealing. Select the Pressure Cook setting at high pressure and set the cook time to 13 minutes. • Once the 13-minute timer has completed and beeps, allow a natural pressure release for 10 minutes and then switch the Pressure Release knob from Sealing to Venting to release any remaining steam. • While the pot is depressurizing, in a small saucepan, bring ⅔ cup of the coconut milk to a simmer over medium heat. Add 5 tbsp of the cane sugar and ¼ tsp of the salt and whisk until the sugar is dissolved and the milk tastes salty-sweet. Keep the sauce warm. • Open the Instant Pot and, with oven mitts, transfer the cooked sticky rice to a large bowl and pour the warm coconut milk mixture on top. Stir well to combine and gently fluff with a fork. Cover and let it sit until the liquid is absorbed, about 20 minutes. You can let the rice rest at room temperature for up to 2 hours. •

Meanwhile, set aside 2 tbsp of the remaining coconut milk in a small bowl. Wipe out the saucepan and add the remaining coconut milk. Add the cornstarch to the small bowl and whisk until smooth, forming a slurry. Bring the coconut milk in the saucepan to a simmer over medium heat, whisking frequently. Whisk the slurry into the coconut milk on the stove and simmer until the mixture has thickened, about 2 minutes. Whisk in the remaining 2 tbsp cane sugar and the remaining ¼ tsp salt until the sugar is dissolved. The coconut cream should be slightly saltier and less sweet than the coconut milk mixture used to cover the rice. • When ready to serve, use a 1-cup measuring cup to scoop the coconut rice into mounds on individual plates and arrange the sliced or diced mango alongside. Drizzle the warm coconut cream over the rice and garnish with the toasted yellow mung beans or sesame seeds. Serve immediately. Do not warm up or refrigerate, as the rice will turn rock hard.

Apple Pie

Ingredients for 6 servings:

3 ½ lb assorted sweet and tart apples 2 tsp lemon juice freshly squeezed 2 tsp ghee ¼ tsp ground cinnamon plus more for serving ⅛ tsp ground allspice ⅛ tsp fine sea salt

Directions and total time – 15-30 min

• **Peel, core, and slice the apples. Place the apples, ¾ cup water, and the lemon juice, ghee, cinnamon, allspice, and salt in an electric pressure cooker. • If using an Instant Pot, secure the lid and turn the valve to pressure. Select the Manual or Pressure Cook button and set it to high pressure for 5 minutes.Once the timer has sounded, let the machine release the pressure on its own; it will take about 15 minutes. (Alternatively, carefully release the pressure manually.) Remove the lid. • Using an immersion blender or conventional blender, pulse the applesauce to your desired consistency. Serve warm with cinnamon sprinkled** on top, or refrigerate and enjoy chilled. ● Store the applesauce in an airtight container in the refrigerator for 10 days or in an airtight container in the freezer for 6 months. Allow it to thaw overnight in the refrigerator before serving. If desired, reheat in a saucepan over medium-low heat for 8 to 10 minutes, until heated through.

Chocolate Yogurt

Ingredients for 12 + servings:

23 oz ultra-filtered chocolate milk like Fairlife 1 tbsp plain or vanilla yogurt with active cultures

Directions and total time – more than 2 hours

• Pour one cup of water in the Instant Pot and insert the steam rack. On the rack place tools that need to be sterilized: a 1-cup glass measure containing a 1 tbsp measure and a heatproof silicone spatula. • Using the display panel select the STEAM function. Use the +/- keys and program the Instant Pot for 3 minutes. • When the time is up, quick-release the pressure. Allow to cool, then remove the tools without touching the inside of the pot or any other surface that will touch food. Drain the pot without touching the inside of the pot. • Using the sterilized tbsp measure, add 1 tbsp of the active-culture yogurt to the sterilized glass measure. Add ⅔ cup of the

milk to the glass measure and use the sterilized spatula to stir until smooth. • Add the remainder of the milk and the yogurt mixture to the pot and use the sterilized spatula to stir until all yogurt is incorporated, then secure the lid, making sure the vent is closed. • Choose the YOGURT function and adjust to the NORMAL or MEDIUM setting. Use the +/- keys and program the Instant Pot for 8 hours. • At the end of the 8 hours, cover the inner pot with plastic wrap and refrigerate at least 8 hours. Do not stir at this point. • At the end of the refrigeration time you will have a pourable chocolate yogurt that pairs wonderfully with fresh berries and granola for a delicious breakfast treat. • To make yogurt pops, pour yogurt mixture into popsicle molds and freeze for at least 8 hours. Unmold and enjoy.

Peanut Butter Cheesecake With Chocolate Crust

Ingredients for 8 Servings:

20 (2-inch) crispy chocolate wafer cookies, or about 1 ⅓ cups chocolate cookie crumbs 1 tablespoon light brown sugar 4 tablespoons unsalted butter, melted ¼ teaspoon fine sea salt ⅔ cup light brown sugar ½ teaspoon fine sea salt 1 tablespoon plus 1 teaspoon cornstarch 16 ounces cream cheese, at room temperature ½ cup plus 2 tablespoons creamy peanut butter (not all-natural) ⅓ cup heavy cream, at room temperature 1 tablespoon pure vanilla extract 2 large eggs, at room temperature Dutch-processed cocoa powder, for dusting

Directions and total time – 5 hours: • **Line the bottom of a 7x3– inch round springform pan with a removable bottom with parchment paper. Lightly spray the sides of the pan with cooking spray or lightly grease with softened butter. • To make the crust, process the cookies in a food processor until finely ground. Add the sugar, melted butter, and salt and** process until combined, scraping the bowl if necessary. Transfer the crumbs to the prepared pan, and using a jar with a flat top on it, press the crumbs down firmly with the upside down jar. Place in the freezer while you prepare the filling. • To make the filling, combine the sugar, salt, and cornstarch in a small bowl and whisk to combine, breaking up any lumps of sugar with your fingers if necessary. • In the bowl of a stand mixer fitted with the paddle attachment, or in a large mixing bowl and using a hand mixer, mix the cream cheese on low until smooth, about 30 seconds to a minute. Slowly add the sugar mixture, stopping the mixer once or twice, and scraping the sides of the bowl with a rubber spatula, until combined, about 1 minute. • Add the peanut butter, heavy cream, and vanilla and mix again until smooth and combined, about 30 seconds to 1 minute. Add the eggs, one at a time, and mix only until combined, scraping the bowl periodically as needed. • Transfer the filling to the prepared pan. Gently drop the pan on the counter a few times to flatten the surface and to pop any air bubbles (it is impossible to pop them all). You may try to smooth the top with a small offset spatula, if you have one, but if you cannot achieve the surface of your dreams, do not fret. • Place 1 cup cold water in the Instant Pot, add the trivet, and place the cheesecake on top of the trivet. Secure the lid and make sure the valve on the top is closed. Push the manual button, and set the timer for 26 minutes on high pressure. The IP will come to pressure almost immediately. • Allow the pot to naturally release, about 20 to 30 minutes. Turn the IP off. Carefully remove the lid, being mindful not to let condensation drip on the cake. However, despite your best efforts, there will be some water on the surface. Use a paper towel to blot it up. • Let the pan cool in the pot until you can easily remove it. Place it on a wire rack and very gently run a paring knife around the edges of the warm cake. Let cool to room temperature. Transfer to the refrigerator and let chill for at least 4 hours, and preferably overnight. • Remove the cake from the sides of pan and with a large spatula, remove the cake from the parchment-lined bottom. Place on a serving platter. Dust with cocoa powder if using, and for clean slices, cut with a large knife dipped in hot water and dried between each cut. The cake will keep refrigerated for up to 3 days. • Some recipes suggest covering the cheesecake in a sheet of paper towel and foil before baking, so as to avoid water on the surface of the cake. But doing so requires you to cook your cheesecake for longer than makes sense to me. I mean, one of the major benefits of baking a cheesecake in an Instant Pot is the speed in which you can do so, not to mention the fact that the water that might accumulate on the surface, once blotted up, has nary an impact on your finished cake.

Triple Citrus Cheesecake

Ingredients for 7 servings:

1 ½ cups graham cracker or vanilla wafer crumbs 2 tablespoons sugar 4 tablespoons melted butter 16 ounces cream cheese, softened ½ cup sugar 1 tablespoon flour ¼ teaspoon salt 2 teaspoons vanilla 2 tablespoons orange juice 2 eggs ½ teaspoon freshly grated lime zest 2 cups water Fresh orange segments (optional)

Directions and total time – 6 hours:

• **Lightly spray a 6-or 7-inch springform pan with cooking spray. Cut a piece of parchment paper to fit the bottom of the pan. Place in the pan and spray again; set aside. • Combine crackers, the 2 tablespoons sugar, and butter in a bowl; mix well. Press into bottom and about 2 inches up the sides of the pan. • In a large bowl beat cream cheese, the ½ cup sugar, flour, salt, vanilla, and orange juice until smooth and creamy. Addeggs, beating just until**

73

combined. Stir in citrus zests. Pour into prepared crust. •
Pour the water into the Instant Pot. Place the trivet in the
bottom of the pot. Cut a piece of foil the same size as a
paper towel. Place the foil under the paper towel and place
the pan on top of the paper towel. Wrap the bottom of the
pan in the foil, with the paper towel as a barrier. • Fold an
18-inch-long piece of foil into thirds lengthwise. Place under
the pan and use the two sides as a sling to place cheesecake
in thepot. Secure the lid on the pot. Close the
pressurerelease valve. • Select manual and cook at high
pressure for 35 minutes. When cooking is complete, use
a natural pressure release to depressurize. • Remove the
cheesecake from the pot using the sling. Cool on a wire rack
for 1 hour and then refrigerate for at least 4 hours.
Carefully remove pan sides. Top cheesecake with fresh
orange segments if desired.

Jalapeño Cheddar Cornbread

Ingredients for 7 servings:

1 cup yellow cornmeal ¾ cup all-purpose flour 2 teaspoons baking powder 2-3 jalapeño peppers seeded and finely chopped, divided 1.25 cups sharp cheddar cheese grated, divided 1 cup fresh or frozen corn ¼ cup green scallions thinly sliced (optional) ¾ cup buttermilk or ¾ cup milk with 1 tsp of lemon juice ¼ cup butter, melted ¼ cup honey 2 eggs, cold 1 teaspoon salt

Directions and total time – 1 hours:

• **Add 1 cup of water to the Instant Pot. Grease and lightly coat 7" cake pan with corn meal and set aside. • In a large mixing bowl, combine the cornmeal, flour, baking powder and salt. Mix well. • Add the grated cheese, chopped jalapeño and scallions (save 1 tablespoon of each to garnish) • Add the corn kernels to the flour mixture. Mix gently until well coated. • In a separate bowl, whisk**

together the buttermilk, melted butter, honey, and eggs. •
Pour over mixed dry ingredients and stir gently with a spoon
until just combined. • Pour into the prepared pan and
garnish with the remaining jalapeño and grated cheese. •
Cover the cake pan with paper towel and aluminum foil.
Place the cake pan on the trivet and gently put the trivet in
the Instant Pot insert. • Cook on Manual(Hi) for 25 minutes
with NPR. You can optionally broil for 2 minutes to
get browned cheese on top. We enjoy the bread as is! •
Enjoy warm.

Thai Red Bean Dessert

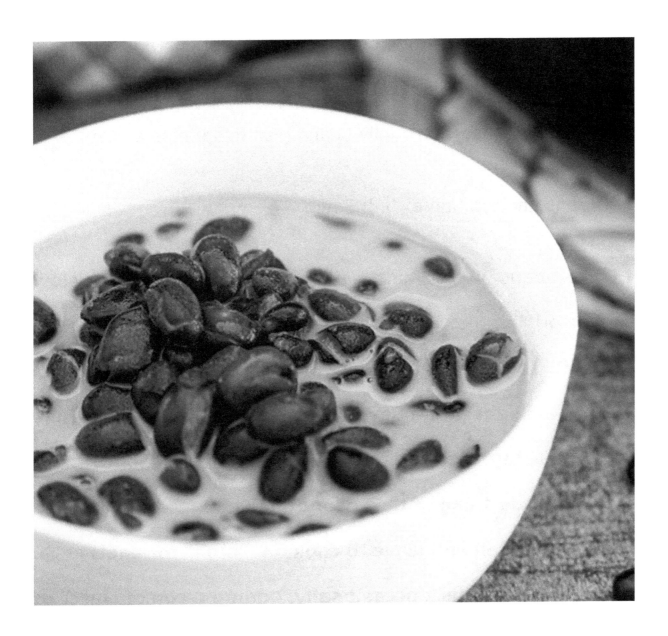

Ingredients for 5 servings:

½ cup beans (red adzuki) 1 ½ cups water 2 cans coconut

milk ½ cup tapioca 2 teaspoons vanilla flavoring ½ cup sugar

(or more depending on desired sweetness) 1 pinch of

salt Optional: 1 handful of dried seaweed Optional: 2

tablespoons coconut (dry shredded baking-type, as is, or

toasted) Optional: a few jelly beans (red to sprinkle on top)

Directions and total time - 2 h 5 min

• **Place beans, water, salt, and seaweed (if using) in a slow**

cooker on "high". Cook for at least 2 hours, or until beans

are soft. If more convenient, leave the beans to cook on

"low" overnight or all day. • Once beans are soft and fully

cooked, using a potato masher, mash beans into small

pieces. • Add 1 can of the coconut milk, sugar, tapioca, and

vanilla. Stir well and leave to cook on "high" for another 30

to 60 minutes. Check occasionally, adding 1 cup of water or

more if the pudding becomes too thick. • Do a taste test

for sweetness and to make sure your tapioca is cooked; it

should no longer taste hard or granular. If using Asian

tapioca, the "pearls" will turn transparent. Regular "minute" tapioca may take slightly longer. • Serve warm in bowls or dessert cups. Top the pudding with some coconut cream to create 2 distinct layers. If desired, add a sprinkling of shredded coconut and a few red jelly beans.

Hot Spiced Fruit

Ingredients for 8 servings:

1 large can (28 to 29 ounces) peach slices (drained) 1 can (8 to 16 ounces) pineapple tidbits with natural juices (undrained) 1 large can (28 to 29 ounces) pear slices (drained) 1 can (15 ounces) mixed chunky fruit ½ cup maraschino cherries (drained) 1 tablespoon cornstarch 1 ½ teaspoons ground cinnamon 1 teaspoon ground nutmeg ½ cup brown sugar 4 tablespoons butter

Directions and total time - 4 h 10 min

• **Combine all ingredients in the slow cooker; stir gently.** • **Cover and cook on LOW for about 4 to 6 hours or on HIGH for 2 to 3 hours.** • **Serve with heavy cream or a dollop of sour cream, if desired.**

Hot Chocolate

Ingredients for 14 servings:

3 cups (about 12 oz.) powdered sugar, sifted 2 cups (about 6 ½ oz.) unsweetened cocoa 6 cups (1 ½ qt.) whole milk 6 cups (1 ½ qt.) half-and-half 2 teaspoons vanilla extract 1 teaspoon kosher salt 1 (10-oz.) pkg. dark chocolate chips (about 1 ½ cups) Toppings: Crushed hard peppermint candies, miniature marshmallows Peppermint schnapps (optional)

Directions and total time - 2 h 15 min

• **Whisk together powdered sugar and cocoa in a 6-quart slow cooker. Turn slow cooker setting to LOW; gradually add milk and half-and-half, whisking constantly to break up lumps. Stir in vanilla and salt; cover and cook until powdered sugar and cocoa are dissolved, about 1 ½ hours. • Uncover slow cooker; add chocolate chips ¼ cup at a time, stirring constantly, until melted, about 2 minutes. Re-cover; continue cooking until mixture thickens,** about 15 minutes. • Serve hot chocolate with peppermint candies, marshmallows, and, if desired, schnapps. Turn slow cooker setting to WARM to hold remaining hot chocolate up to 2 hours.

Plimoth Plantation Indian Pudding

Ingredients for 3 servings:

3 c whole milk ½ c cornmeal ½ teaspoon table salt 2 tablespoons unsalted butter, plus extra for greasing cooker 2 large eggs ⅓ c molasses 1 teaspoon cinnamon ½ teaspoon ginger ½ c dried cranberries (optional)

Directions and total time - 2 h 20 min

• **Grease inside of your slow cooker with butter and preheat on high for 15 minutes.** • **In a large heavy-bottom pot, whisk together milk, cornmeal, and salt and bring to a boil. Continue whisking another 5 minutes; then cover and simmer on low 10 minutes. Remove from burner and add butter. In a medium size bowl, combine eggs, molasses, and spices.** • **Add some of the hot cornmeal mixture to the egg mixture to temper the eggs; then transfer egg mixture into the pot. Stir in cranberries, if you like. Scrape batter into the slow cooker and cook on high 2 to 3 hours or on low 6-8**

hours. The center will be not quite set. Serve warm topped with ice cream, whipped cream, or light cream.

Apples and Apricots Confiture

Ingredients for 10 servings:

500 g Apples 500 g Apricots 500 g Sugar 1 glass Water

Directions and total time - 2 h 20 min • Cut the skin from apples, but do not discard. Pour it with a glass of boiling water, place in the bowl of the slow cooker and steam in the "Steam cooking" mode for 10 minutes. This will release pectin from them, which will give perfect condensation to the future jam. • Catch the peel with a slotted spoon, and leave the liquid from it in the bowl. • Cut apples and put in the bowl of the device. Washed, seedless fruits apricots are ground in any convenient way. Spread fruit puree in a saucepan in layers, pouring sugar. • Cover the appliance with a lid and set the "Extinguishing" mode. Leave to languish for an hour. • Open the lid and mix the resulting mass. Be sure to wipe the lid from condensation. • Close the appliance again and set the "Baking" mode for 40 minutes. Do not close the lid tightly; in the process of languishing, mix the jam a couple of times. •

Traditionally, lay the finished jam in sterilized jars and close it

tightly.

Chocolate Lava Cake

Ingredients for 8 servings:

Cake Mixture 2 cups plain flour 1 cup sugar 1 tablespoon baking powder ⅓ cup cocoa powder 1 teaspoon salt ¼ cup unsalted butter, melted 1 tsp vanilla extract 1 cup milk Chocolate "Lava" Sauce 1 cup brown sugar ½ cup unsweetened cocoa powder 3 cups boiling water

Directions and total time - 4 h 20 min

• **Lightly grease the slow cooker with butter or oil. • In a bowl, combine the flour, sugar, baking powder, cocoa powder, and salt. • Make a well in the middle and pour in the melted butter, vanilla, and milk. • Stir until well combined. • Pour into the slow cooker. • In another bowl, combine the brown sugar and cocoa powder. Sprinkle this mixture over the cake mixture. • Gently pour the boiling water over the top. • Place the lid on and cook on low for 3-4 hours or until the cake is cooked.**

Raspberry Upside-Down Cake

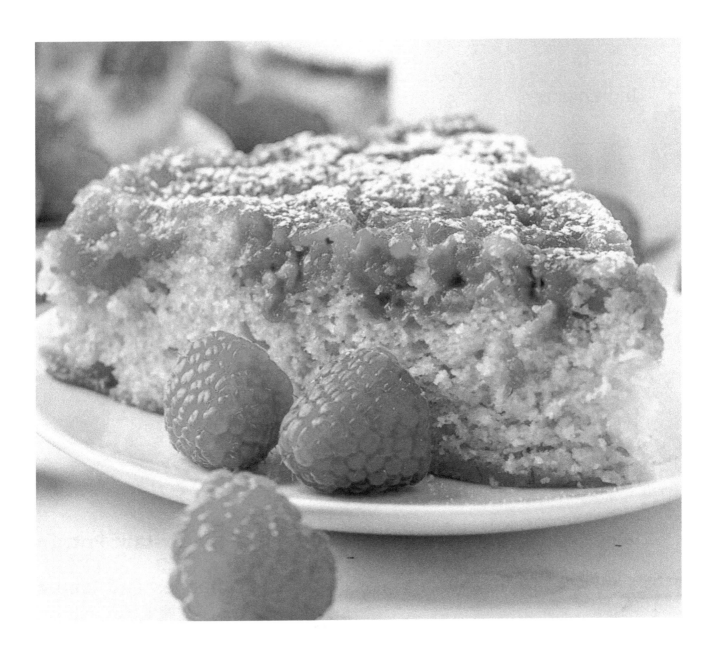

(Ready in about 35 minutes | Servings 5)

Per serving: 193 Calories; 17.9g Fat; 9.1g Carbs; 1.2g Protein; 3.4g Sugars

Ingredients

1/2 pound raspberries 1 ½ tablespoons lemon juice 1 cup coconut flour 2 tablespoons cassava flour 1/2 teaspoon baking powder 1/8 teaspoon sea salt 1/4 cup coconut oil, melted 1 tablespoon monk fruit powder 1/2 teaspoon ground cinnamon 1/4 teaspoon grated nutmeg 1/2 teaspoon orange zest 1 teaspoon vanilla paste 1 ½ teaspoons powdered agar

Directions

Add 1 ½ cups water and a metal rack to the Instant Pot. In a mixing bowl, thoroughly combine raspberries and lemon juice. Spread raspberries in the bottom of the pan. In another mixing bowl, thoroughly combine coconut flour, cassava flour, baking powder, and sea salt. In the third

bowl, mix the coconut oil, monk fruit powder, cinnamon, nutmeg, orange zest, and vanilla. Add powdered agar and mix until everything is well incorporated. Pour the liquid ingredients over dry ingredients and mix to form a dough; flatten it to form a circle. Place this dough in a baking pan and cover the raspberries. Cover the pan with a sheet of aluminum foil. Lower the pan onto the metal rack. Secure the lid. Choose "Manual" mode and High pressure; cook for 27 minutes. Once cooking is complete, use a natural pressure release; carefully remove the lid. Finally, turn the cake pan upside down and unmold it on a platter. Enjoy!

Grandma's Orange Cheesecake

(Ready in about 35 minutes + chilling time | Servings 10)

Per serving: 188 Calories; 17.2g Fat; 4.5g Carbs; 5.5g Protein; 1.3g Sugars

Ingredients

Crust: 1/2 cup almond flour 1/2 cup coconut flour 1 ½ tablespoons powdered erythritol 1/4 teaspoon kosher salt 3 tablespoons butter, melted Filling: 8 ounces sour cream, at room temperature 8 ounces cream cheese, at room temperature 1/2 cup powdered erythritol 3 tablespoons orange juice 1/2 teaspoon ginger powder 1 teaspoon vanilla extract 3 eggs, at room temperature

Directions

Line a round baking pan with a piece of parchment paper. In a mixing bowl, thoroughly combine all crust ingredients

in the order listed above. Press the crust mixture into the bottom of the pan. Then, make the filling by mixing the sour cream and cream cheese until uniform and smooth; add the remaining ingredients and continue to beat until everything is well combined. Pour the cream cheese mixture over the crust. Cover with aluminum foil, making a foil sling. Place 1 ½ cups of water and a metal trivet in your Instant Pot. Then, place the pan on the metal rack. Secure the lid. Choose "Manual" mode and High pressure; cook for 30 minutes. Once cooking is complete, use a natural pressure release; carefully remove the lid. Serve well chilled and enjoy!

Yummy and Easy Chocolate Mousse

(Ready in about 20 minutes + chilling time | Servings 6)

Per serving: 205 Calories; 18.3g Fat; 9.2g Carbs; 3.2g Protein; 6.6g Sugars

Ingredients

1 cup full-fat milk 1 cup heavy cream 4 egg yolks, beaten 1/3 cup sugar 1/4 teaspoon grated nutmeg 1/4 teaspoon ground cinnamon 1/4 cup unsweetened cocoa powder

Directions

In a small pan, bring the milk and cream to a simmer. In a mixing dish, thoroughly combine the remaining ingredients. Add this egg mixture to the warm milk mixture. Pour the mixture into ramekins. Add 1 ½ cups of water and a metal rack to the Instant Pot. Now, lower your ramekins onto the rack. Secure the lid. Choose "Manual" mode and High

pressure; cook for 10 minutes. Once cooking is complete, use a natural pressure release; carefully remove the lid. Serve Serve well chilled and enjoy!

Almond and Chocolate Crème

(Ready in about 15 minutes | Servings 4)

Per serving: 401 Calories; 37.1g Fat; 9.2g Carbs; 9.1g Protein; 2.7g Sugars

Ingredients

2 cups heavy whipping cream 1/2 cup water 4 eggs 1/3 cup Swerve 1 teaspoon almond extract 1 teaspoon vanilla extract 1/3 cup almonds, ground 2 tablespoons coconut oil, room temperature 4 tablespoons cacao powder 2 tablespoons gelatin

Directions

Start by adding 1 ½ cups of water and a metal rack to your Instant Pot. Blend the cream, water, eggs, Swerve, almond extract, vanilla extract and almonds in your food processor. Add the remaining ingredients and process for a minute longer. Divide the mixture between four Mason jars; cover

your jars with lids. Lower the jars onto the rack. Secure the lid. Choose "Manual" mode and High pressure; cook for 7 minutes. Once cooking is complete, use a natural pressure release; carefully remove the lid. Bon appétit!

Navel Orange Cheesecake

(Ready in about 30 minutes + chilling time | Servings 5)

Per serving: 268 Calories; 22.7g Fat; 6.6g Carbs; 9.5g Protein; 5.2g Sugars

Ingredients

9 ounces cream cheese 1/3 cup Swerve 1/2 teaspoon ginger powder 1 teaspoon grated orange zest 1 teaspoon vanilla extract 3 eggs 4 tablespoons double cream 1 tablespoon Swerve 1 navel orange, peeled and sliced

Directions

Start by adding 1 ½ cups of water and a metal rack to your Instant Pot. Now, spritz a baking pan with a nonstick cooking spray. Beat cream cheese, 1/3 cup of Swerve, ginger, grated orange zest, and vanilla with an electric mixer. Now, gradually fold in the eggs, and continue to mix

until everything is well incorporated. Press this mixture into the prepared baking pan and cover with foil. Secure the lid. Choose "Bean/Chili" mode and High pressure; cook for 25 minutes. Once cooking is complete, use a natural pressure release; carefully remove the lid. Mix the cream and 1 tablespoon of Swerve; spread this topping on the cake. Allow it to cool on a wire rack. Then, transfer your cake to the refrigerator. Garnish with orange slices and serve well chilled. Bon appétit!

Fabulous Blackberry Brownies

(Ready in about 30 minutes | Servings 8)

Per serving: 151 Calories; 13.6g Fat; 6.7g Carbs; 4.1g Protein; 1.1g Sugars

Ingredients

4 eggs 1 ¼ cups coconut cream 1 teaspoon Stevia liquid concentrate 1/3 cup cocoa powder, unsweetened 1/2 teaspoon grated nutmeg 1/2 teaspoon cinnamon powder 1 teaspoon espresso coffee 1 teaspoon pure almond extract 1 teaspoon pure vanilla extract 1 teaspoon baking powder A pinch of kosher salt 1 cup blackberries, fresh or frozen (thawed)

Instructions

Start by adding 1 ½ cups of water and a metal rack to your Instant Pot. Now, spritz a baking pan with a nonstick cooking spray. Now, mix eggs, coconut cream, Stevia, cocoa

powder, nutmeg, cinnamon, coffee, pure almond extract vanilla, baking powder, and salt with an electric mixer. Crush the blackberries with a fork. After that, fold in your blackberries into the prepared mixture. Pour the batter into the prepared pan. Secure the lid. Choose "Bean/Chili" mode and High pressure; cook for 25 minutes. Once cooking is complete, use a natural pressure release; carefully remove the lid. Bon appétit!

Coconut and Lemon Squares

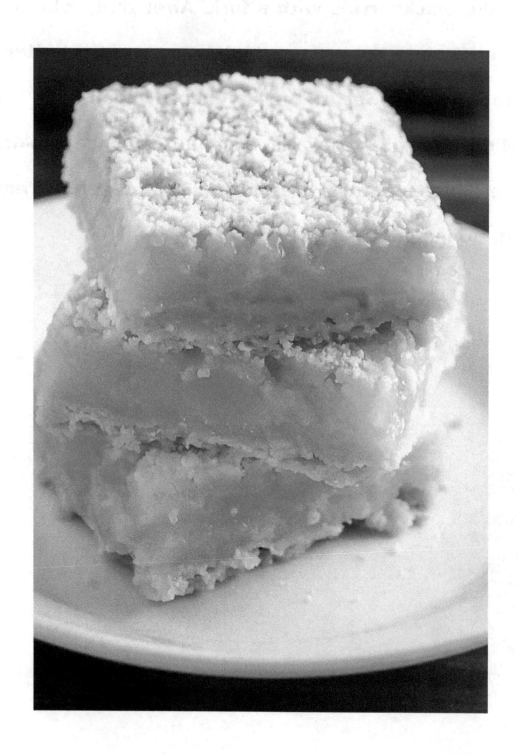

(Ready in about 25 minutes | Servings 6)

Per serving: 173 Calories; 15.6g Fat; 2.5g Carbs; 6.2g Protein; 1.6g Sugars

Ingredients

Crust: 3/4 cup coconut flour 1/4 cup coconut oil 2 tablespoons Swerve 1/2 teaspoon pure lemon extract 1/2 teaspoon pure coconut extract 1/2 teaspoon pure vanilla extract 1/2 teaspoon baking powder A pinch of grated nutmeg A pinch of salt Filling: 4 eggs 1/2 cup Swerve 3 tablespoons freshly squeezed lemon juice 3 tablespoons shredded coconut 1/4 teaspoon cinnamon powder

Directions

Start by adding 1 ½ cups of water and a metal rack to your Instant Pot. Now, spritz a baking pan with a nonstick cooking spray (butter flavor). Then, thoroughly combine all crust ingredients in your food processor. Now, spread the

crust mixture evenly on the bottom of the prepared pan. Do not forget to prick a few holes with a fork. Lower the baking pan onto the rack. Secure the lid. Choose "Manual" mode and High pressure; cook for 8 minutes. Once cooking is complete, use a quick pressure release; carefully remove the lid. Meanwhile, thoroughly combine all filling ingredients in your food processor. Spread the filling mixture evenly over top of the warm crust. Return to the Instant Pot. Secure the lid. Choose "Manual" mode and High pressure; cook for 15 minutes. Once cooking is complete, use a quick pressure release; carefully remove the lid. Cut into squares and serve at room temperature or chilled. Bon appétit!

Sophisticated Lavender Brownies

(Ready in about 30 minutes | Servings 6)

Per serving: 384 Calories; 36.6g Fat; 7.2g Carbs; 7.7g Protein; 1.3g Sugars

Ingredients

4 ounces chocolate, sugar-free 1/2 cup coconut oil 2 cups Swerve 4 eggs, whisked 1 teaspoon vanilla paste 1/4 teaspoon sea salt 1/4 teaspoon grated nutmeg 1/2 teaspoon dried lavender flowers 1/4 cup almond flour 1/2 cup whipped cream

Directions **Start by adding 1 ½ cups of water and a metal trivet to your Instant Pot. Now, spritz a baking pan with a nonstick cooking spray. Thoroughly combine the chocolate, coconut oil, and Swerve. Gradually, whisk in the eggs. Add the vanilla paste, salt, nutmeg, lavender flowers and almond flour; mix until everything is well incorporated. Secure the lid. Choose "Bean/Chili" mode and High** pressure; cook for 25 minutes. Once cooking is complete, use a natural pressure release; carefully remove the lid. Top with whipped cream and serve well chilled. Bon appétit!

Coconut and Raspberry Cupcakes

(Ready in about 35 minutes | Servings 6)

Per serving: 403 Calories; 42.1g Fat; 4.1g Carbs; 4.2g Protein; 2.1g Sugars

Ingredients

Cupcakes: 1/2 cup coconut flour 1/2 cup almond flour 1/2 teaspoon baking soda 1 teaspoon baking powder A pinch of salt A pinch of grated nutmeg 1 teaspoon ginger powder 1 stick butter, at room temperature 1/2 cup Swerve 3 eggs, beaten 1/2 teaspoon pure coconut extract 1/2 teaspoon pure vanilla extract 1/2 cup double cream Frosting: 1 stick butter, at room temperature 1/2 cup Swerve 1 teaspoon pure vanilla extract 1/2 teaspoon coconut extract 6 tablespoons coconut, shredded 3 tablespoons raspberry, puréed 6 frozen raspberries

Directions

Start by adding 1 ½ cups of water and a rack to your Instant Pot. In a mixing dish, thoroughly combine the cupcake ingredients. Divide the batter between silicone cupcake liners. Cover with a piece of foil. Place the cupcakes on the rack. Secure the lid. Choose "Manual" mode and High pressure; cook for 25 minutes. Once cooking is complete, use a natural pressure release; carefully remove the lid. In the meantime, thoroughly combine the frosting ingredients. Put this mixture into a piping bag and top your cupcakes. Garnish with frozen raspberries and enjoy!

Conclusion

Did you appreciate attempting these brand-new and also tasty dishes?

Regrettably we have come to the end of this recipe book relating to the use of the fantastic Ninja Foodi multi-cooker, which I really wish you enjoyed.

To improve your health we would love to advise you to combine exercise as well as a dynamic way of living along with following these fantastic recipes, so as to highlight the enhancements. we will be back quickly with increasingly more fascinating vegetarian dishes, a large hug, see you soon.

CPSIA information can be obtained
at www.ICGtesting.com
Printed in the USA
LVHW062315230521
688301LV00007B/349

9 781667 103990